Awakening with Ayahuasca: A Journey to Healing, Wisdom, and Transformation

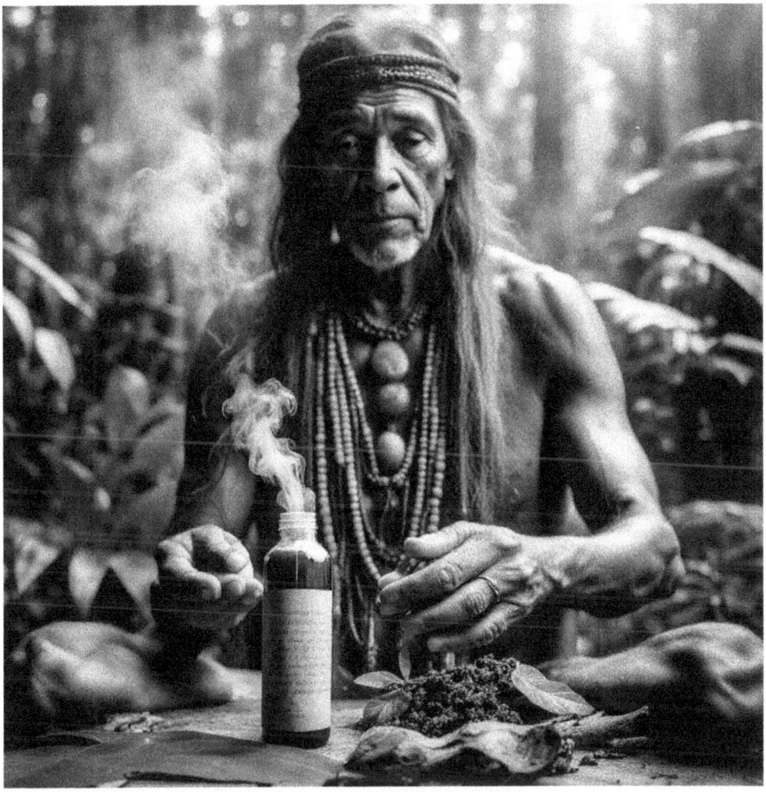

Introduction

Ayahuasca, an ancient Amazonian brew, has garnered significant attention in recent years for its potential therapeutic and transformative properties. In this comprehensive study, we'll delve into the history, benefits, risks, and cultural significance of Ayahuasca. Our aim is to provide an honest and well-rounded view while incorporating advanced SEO techniques to enhance your experience and that of others.

Table of Contents

- The potential future of Ayahuasca in mainstream medicine.

Bonus

- Shamanic Empowerment with Ayahuasca Herself
- Meet the 3 Elders keepers of sacred knowledge
- Shamanic guided meditation with ayahuasca and her Healings
- A journey together with the Author in one of his favourites Ayahuasca out of body experience
- Protection and empowerment of the blue macaw, Bobinsana mermaid and the White Eagle in a shamanic transmission that will bless you for a lifetime

---

In this comprehensive article, we'll explore Ayahuasca from various angles, aiming to provide valuable insights for those interested in understanding its history, effects, and potential benefits, all while emphasizing the importance of responsible use and respecting its cultural context.

About The Author:

Thiago Soares Zaupa, a luminary seeker and guardian of ancient wisdom, has ventured deep into the heart of the Amazon, where the rainforest's vibrant pulse resonates with the songs of medicinal plants. Over the span of eight transformative years, he devoted himself to the sacred art of medicinal plants and plant diets—an odyssey that imbued his spirit with profound understanding.

In the emerald tapestry of the jungle, he meticulously honed his craft, emerging as a master in the sacred arts of Ayahuasca, San Pedro, and Bobinsana. Under their benevolent guidance, he unlocked the doorways to profound healing and transformation, sharing their gifts with those who sought his wisdom.

He is not merely a shaman but a healer, tenderly guiding others on their soul's journey, unveiling the hidden tapestries of their own hearts. He has witnessed the alchemical miracles that can transpire in the mystical embrace of Ayahuasca, providing solace, illumination, and rejuvenation.

He have contributed to the healing shamanic community with numerous valuable books, information, researches and sacred healing songs.

His journey doesn't end there. He is a dedicated yogi, melding the physical and the metaphysical through the ancient art of yoga. The balance he finds on his mat reverberates in every aspect of his life, and he gracefully weaves this harmony into his sacred work.

Discipline is his steadfast companion. He has delved into the world of over 200 master plants, understanding their unique characters and how they can heal the body, mind, and spirit. His commitment led him to establish a healing center in the heart of the Amazon, a sanctuary where others can safely embrace their own sacred transformations.

Today he lives in Europe with his family, his wife a valuable herbalist and knower of the arts of healing using all types of different medicinal herbs, mixtures, ayurvedic recipes and energy work such as advanced reiki and theta healing that can be used as alternative practices for different types of treatments and healings on the energetic core, mental and spiritual level.

Meditation is his sanctuary, a space where he explores the depths of consciousness. From Buddhist meditations to other ancient practices, he has mastered the art of stillness and profound contemplation.

In the symphony of life, he is also a musician, drawing on the rhythms of the Amazon and the melodies of his heart. His music is an offering, a sacred bridge to the spirits and a gift to those who walk alongside him on this path.

He is a keeper of tradition, the thread that connects the ancient to the modern. His journey is a testament to the timeless wisdom of the Amazon and nature herself, a testament to the power of healing, and a testament to the profound potential of the human spirit.

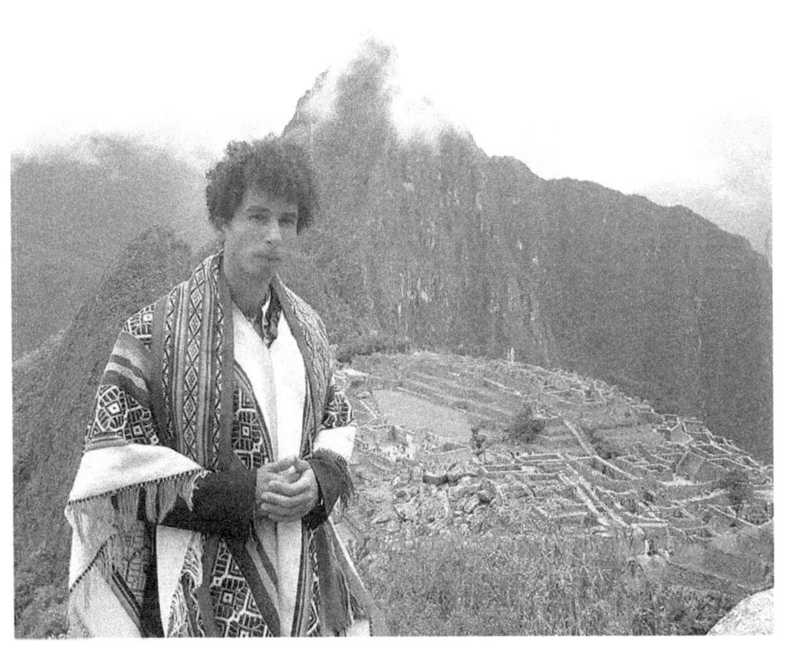

What is Ayahuasca?
- **A brief introduction to Ayahuasca.**

Ayahuasca is a powerful psychoactive plant medicine with a long history of traditional use among indigenous people in the Amazon rainforest. It is known for its potent hallucinogenic and healing properties. Ayahuasca is typically prepared as a brew or tea by combining two main plant ingredients: the Banisteriopsis caapi vine and the leaves of the Psychotria viridis shrub. These two plants contain compounds that, when combined, create a brew that induces profound altered states of consciousness.

The active compounds in Ayahuasca are primarily dimethyltryptamine (DMT) from the Psychotria viridis leaves and harmine, harmaline, and tetrahydroharmine from the Banisteriopsis caapi vine. DMT is a powerful psychedelic compound that, when ingested orally, would normally be broken down by enzymes in the digestive system. However, the harmala alkaloids in the Banisteriopsis caapi vine act as inhibitors of these enzymes, allowing DMT to be absorbed and produce its psychedelic effects.

Ayahuasca has been used for centuries in indigenous shamanic rituals as a means of gaining insights, healing, and connecting with the spirit world. In recent years, it has gained popularity in the Western world as a tool for personal and spiritual growth, as well as for its potential therapeutic benefits. Some people use Ayahuasca to explore their consciousness, confront unresolved emotional issues, and seek profound insights into their lives.

It's important to note that Ayahuasca is a potent substance and should be used with caution. It can induce intense and often challenging experiences, sometimes referred to as "the purge," which can include vomiting and diarrhea. These experiences are seen as part of the healing process in traditional Amazonian practices.

The use of Ayahuasca has also raised legal and ethical concerns, as it contains controlled substances in many countries. In some places, there is a growing movement to legalize or decriminalize Ayahuasca for religious or therapeutic use. If you are considering trying Ayahuasca, it is essential to do thorough research, consult with experienced practitioners, and ensure you are in a safe and supportive environment.

- **The origin and history of Ayahuasca use.**

The origin and history of Ayahuasca use is deeply intertwined with the indigenous cultures of the Amazon rainforest in South America. It has been an integral part of their spiritual and healing traditions for centuries. Here's an overview of the origin and history of Ayahuasca use:

Origin:

Ayahuasca's precise origin is challenging to pinpoint due to its long history and the diverse range of indigenous tribes in the Amazon region. It is believed to have emerged in the western Amazon basin, in areas that now encompass modern-day Peru, Ecuador, Brazil, and Colombia. The name "Ayahuasca" is derived from two Quechua words: "aya," meaning spirit, and "huasca," meaning vine. This name reflects the central role of the Ayahuasca vine in indigenous shamanic practices, where it is considered a conduit to the spirit world.

Historical Use:

The use of Ayahuasca dates back at least a few centuries, with some estimates suggesting that it could have been in use for over a thousand years. It is closely tied to the spiritual and healing practices of various indigenous tribes, including the Shipibo, the Shuar, the Quechua, and the Ayahuasca people, among others.

Indigenous shamans or healers, known as "ayahuasqueros" or "curanderos," have traditionally brewed and administered Ayahuasca in rituals and ceremonies. These rituals often involve singing traditional icaros (healing songs), chanting, and invoking the spirit world to gain insights, heal ailments, and connect with the plants and animals of the rainforest.

Spread to the Western World:

Ayahuasca remained largely unknown outside of indigenous communities until the mid-20th century. The first recorded encounter of Ayahuasca by a Westerner was in 1851 by a British botanist named Richard Spruce. However, it wasn't until the mid-20th century that Ayahuasca began to attract the attention of Western researchers and spiritual seekers.

In the 1960s and 1970s, Ayahuasca gained prominence in the counterculture movement, with figures like Terence McKenna and Dennis McKenna advocating for its exploration. This led to an increased interest in Ayahuasca's potential for personal growth and healing, and it began to spread beyond the Amazon region.

Modern Ayahuasca Use:

Today, Ayahuasca has gained global recognition for its potential therapeutic and spiritual benefits. It is used in various contexts, including shamanic retreats, religious ceremonies, and therapeutic settings. Some countries, like Brazil and Peru, have established legal frameworks to regulate and support the use of Ayahuasca, especially within religious practices.

However, the global popularity of Ayahuasca has also raised concerns about cultural appropriation, sustainability, and the need to preserve the traditional knowledge and practices of indigenous communities.

The history of Ayahuasca is a complex tapestry that encompasses indigenous wisdom, Western exploration, and ongoing debates about its cultural and legal significance. It continues to be a subject of fascination, research, and debate in the modern world.

The Ayahuasca Experience
- **Detailed insights into the Ayahuasca journey.**

Embarking on the Enchanted Journey:

As one delicately sips the sacred elixir of Ayahuasca, a sense of eager anticipation fills the air. These initial moments are akin to the opening of a mystical doorway, gently beckoning us toward the threshold of an enigmatic world. Our surroundings start to blur, and the boundaries that define our self begin to gracefully dissolve.

Unveiling the Psychedelic Tapestry:

With closed eyes, the mind unfurls like a vibrant tapestry adorned with kaleidoscopic visions and vivid dreams. Intricate patterns dance in radiant hues, weaving together the fabric of our perceptions and hinting at the interconnectedness of all things.

Each sound, scent, and touch takes on a heightened significance as the senses awaken to their fullest potential.

Voyage into the Subconscious:

The Ayahuasca journey is a profound odyssey into the depths of our subconscious, where hidden memories, unspoken emotions, and long-buried fears gently rise to the surface. It serves as a mirror to the soul, reflecting our innermost landscape with unparalleled clarity. In this sacred space, we may confront our deepest fears and traumas, allowing for profound healing and catharsis.

Conversations with the Spirit Realm:

A profound sense of oneness with the cosmos envelops the Ayahuasca experience, as if one is in communion with ethereal entities, ancient plant spirits, or ancestral guardians. These otherworldly encounters provide profound insights, guidance, and an overwhelming sense of reverence for the profound mysteries of existence.

The Purification and Renewal:

Ayahuasca is renowned for its purgative qualities, which may include moments of cleansing through vomiting or diarrhea. This facet of the journey, often referred to as "the purge," symbolizes the necessary release of physical and emotional toxins. It is a transformative act of shedding what no longer serves us, leaving a profound sensation of lightness and renewal.

Timelessness and Eternity:

In the realm of Ayahuasca, the constraints of time gently dissolve, and one may lose themselves in the eternal present. It is a space where past and future merge, inviting a deep exploration of self and universe, liberated from the rigidity of linear time.

Integration and Metamorphosis:

As the Ayahuasca journey gracefully draws to a close, we find ourselves guided back to the material world. The insights acquired, the wounds tenderly healed, and the wisdom gently gathered become cherished gifts to be carried into the tapestry of our daily lives. This transformation is an ongoing process, requiring patience and introspection to fully integrate.
As the ceremonial journey comes to an end, another one commences - the everyday ceremony of life, integrating the newfound wisdom and insights into our daily existence. It's an opportunity to respond to the former self in a new way. This transformation is a gradual process that demands patience and a genuine

willingness to change. When approached with these qualities, the lasting effects of the ceremony become an enduring and transformative part of one's life.

The Ayahuasca experience is a voyage of profound wonder, insight, and rebirth, offering glimpses into the interconnectedness of existence and the boundless potential of the human spirit. It is a transformative journey that inspires profound change and leads us toward a deeper understanding of self, the universe, and the infinite enigmas that lie beyond.

- **Common experiences and effects.**

The Ayahuasca experience can vary from person to person, but there are some common experiences and effects that many individuals report during their journeys. These effects include both the physical and psychological aspects of the Ayahuasca experience:

1. Vomiting and Purging: Many Ayahuasca ceremonies involve purging, which can include vomiting and, less commonly, diarrhea. This is often seen as a form of cleansing and is referred to as "the purge." However, the purge should not be feared; it is a natural process during the ceremony. What once felt heavy and limiting will suddenly become light and liberating. Embracing the purge through surrender, trust, and letting go will lead to a profound sense of well-being, transforming your Ayahuasca journey into a life-changing experience.

2. Visual and Sensory Hallucinations: Ayahuasca can induce intense visual and sensory experiences. Users often report seeing intricate and colorful geometric patterns, as well as vivid images and scenes. These hallucinations are often described as both beautiful and awe-inspiring. While the visionary effects can be profound, one should not be disheartened if they don't experience vibrant, colorful visions. The plant spirit possesses intelligence, tailoring the healing ceremony to individual requirements. Whether or not visions manifest, the healing process unfolds regardless.

3. Altered Perception of Time: Time can become distorted during an Ayahuasca journey. It may feel like minutes stretch into hours or that you've experienced a lifetime in the span of a single ceremony. Enveloped by the Great Spirit of Mother Ayahuasca, time loses its significance, and everything unfolds in the present moment. Nothing else holds importance.

4. Emotional Release: Ayahuasca can bring repressed emotions and memories to the surface. This can lead to intense emotional experiences, including both catharsis and the release of trauma. Certain memories may evoke the sensation of being in the present moment, making them more difficult to observe. It is crucial to cultivate profound trust in the plant and the entire process, allowing these emotions to flow freely and embracing them. By doing so, one can welcome a profound sense of liberation and release that permeates their entire being.

5. Spiritual Insights: Many users report profound spiritual or metaphysical insights during their Ayahuasca experiences. They may feel a deep sense of interconnectedness with all of existence and encounter entities or beings in the spirit world.

6. Self-Reflection and Self-Exploration: Ayahuasca often prompts deep self-reflection. Users may gain new perspectives on their lives, behavior, and relationships, which can lead to personal growth and healing.

7. Increased Sensitivity: People often become more sensitive to their surroundings, emotions, and bodily sensations. They may feel a heightened sense of empathy and connection to nature. Also, in this state, they become more attuned to their own needs and the energies surrounding them, gaining a deeper understanding of what truly brings them happiness. Often, the Spirit of the plant assists in opening the heart, fostering a sense of gratitude and compassion within.

8. Ego Dissolution: Ayahuasca can lead to the dissolution of one's ego or sense of self, which can be a profound and sometimes challenging experience. This dissolution can lead to a sense of oneness with the universe.

9. Integration and Insight: After the ceremony, many users report that they gain new insights and a deeper understanding of their experiences. These insights can be transformative and can guide personal growth and change.

It's important to note that not all Ayahuasca experiences are the same, and individual reactions can vary widely. The effects can be influenced by factors such as the dose, the individual's mental and emotional state, the setting, and the expertise of the facilitator or shaman guiding the ceremony. Additionally, while Ayahuasca can be a powerful tool for healing and personal growth, it can also be mentally and emotionally challenging. It should be approached with respect, preparation, and under the guidance of experienced individuals in a safe and supportive environment.

Health Benefits of Ayahuasca
- **A discussion of the potential therapeutic benefits.**

Ayahuasca is increasingly being explored for its potential therapeutic benefits, although it's important to note that research in this area is still in its early stages. While the effects of Ayahuasca can vary widely among individuals, there is a growing body of anecdotal evidence and some preliminary scientific research suggesting that it may have therapeutic potential in several areas:

1. Mental Health and Well-Being:

- Depression and Anxiety: Some studies and anecdotal reports suggest that Ayahuasca may offer relief from symptoms of depression and anxiety. It is believed to promote introspection and emotional processing, potentially leading to a reduction in these symptoms.
- Post-Traumatic Stress Disorder (PTSD): Ayahuasca-assisted therapy is being explored as a potential treatment for individuals with PTSD. It may help patients confront and process traumatic experiences in a controlled and supportive environment.

2. Addiction Treatment:

- Substance Use Disorders: Ayahuasca has been studied as a potential treatment for addiction, including alcohol and drug dependencies. Some individuals report that Ayahuasca experiences lead to a shift in their relationship with addictive substances.

3. Personal Growth and Self-Exploration:

- Spiritual Insights: Many people who use Ayahuasca report profound spiritual experiences and insights. These insights may contribute to personal growth, self-discovery, and a greater sense of purpose.
- Enhanced Creativity and Problem Solving: Ayahuasca experiences can lead to enhanced creativity and improved problem-solving abilities. Some individuals find it helpful for breaking through creative blocks.

4. Psychospiritual Healing:

- Resolution of Past Traumas: Ayahuasca ceremonies often involve emotional catharsis, which may facilitate the resolution of past traumas and emotional wounds. Frequently, this grants the ability to view situations from a different perspective, making it easier to understand, forgive, and ultimately let go.
- Connection and Unity: The sense of interconnectedness and unity experienced during Ayahuasca ceremonies can have a positive impact on one's perception of the self and others, potentially promoting empathy and compassion.

5. Palliative Care and End-of-Life Anxiety:

- Terminal Illness: Ayahuasca is being explored as a means of providing comfort and addressing existential distress for individuals facing terminal illness. It may help individuals come to terms with mortality and find peace.

It's important to emphasize that Ayahuasca is not a guaranteed or standardized treatment for any specific condition, and it should not be considered a replacement for conventional medical or psychological therapies. Its use should always be guided by experienced practitioners in controlled, safe settings.

Furthermore, Ayahuasca is not without risks, and adverse reactions are possible, particularly when not used responsibly. Potential side effects and contraindications, such as interactions with certain medications or pre-existing health conditions, need to be carefully considered.

The exploration of Ayahuasca's therapeutic potential is a rapidly evolving field, and ongoing research will be instrumental in establishing its safety and efficacy as a complementary therapy for various mental and emotional health conditions. It is advisable for individuals interested in Ayahuasca therapy to seek guidance from trained professionals and participate in controlled, legal, and ethical settings.

- **Research on Ayahuasca and mental health.**

Research on Ayahuasca and mental health is a growing field, and while it is still in its early stages, there is increasing interest in understanding the potential therapeutic effects of this plant medicine on various mental health conditions. Here are some key areas of research and findings related to Ayahuasca and mental health:

1. Depression and Anxiety:

- A study published in the journal "Psychopharmacology" in 2016 found that Ayahuasca may lead to significant and sustained improvements in the symptoms of depression and anxiety. Participants reported a decrease in depressive symptoms that lasted for several weeks after the Ayahuasca experience.

2. Post-Traumatic Stress Disorder (PTSD):

- Research is ongoing, but early studies and anecdotal reports suggest that Ayahuasca-assisted therapy may help individuals with PTSD confront and process traumatic memories. The ceremonies' therapeutic setting and the emotional release that often occurs during the experience may be conducive to addressing PTSD symptoms.

3. Addiction Treatment:

- A 2013 study published in the "Journal of Psychoactive Drugs" explored Ayahuasca's potential as a treatment for substance use disorders. The results suggested that Ayahuasca may have the potential to facilitate abstinence from addictive substances and lead to insights into the root causes of addiction.

4. Personal Growth and Well-Being:

- Research has shown that Ayahuasca experiences are often associated with enhanced feelings of personal growth, self-exploration, and an improved sense of well-being. Many participants report that they gain a greater understanding of themselves and their life's purpose.

5. Spirituality and Quality of Life:

- Ayahuasca is often associated with spiritual experiences, and these experiences can positively influence an individual's sense of meaning, purpose, and overall quality of life.

6. Palliative Care:

- Ayahuasca has been explored as a means of providing comfort and addressing existential distress for individuals with terminal illnesses. It may help individuals come to terms with mortality and find peace as they approach the end of life.

It's important to note that the research on Ayahuasca and mental health is still limited, and more rigorous clinical trials are needed to establish its safety and efficacy for specific mental health conditions. Furthermore, Ayahuasca is a powerful substance and should only be used under the guidance of experienced facilitators in controlled, safe, and legal settings.

Additionally, regulatory and legal considerations vary by country, so it's essential to be aware of the local regulations and guidelines regarding Ayahuasca use for mental health or therapeutic purposes. If you or someone you know is considering Ayahuasca for mental health reasons, it is crucial to consult with healthcare professionals and experienced practitioners to make informed and responsible choices.

Risks and Precautions
- **Addressing the potential risks and contraindications.**

Ayahuasca is a potent and sacred plant medicine, and like any powerful substance, it carries potential risks and contraindications. It should be approached with caution and responsibility. Here are some important considerations regarding the risks and precautions associated with Ayahuasca:

1. Psychological Vulnerability:

- Individuals with a history of severe mental health conditions, such as schizophrenia or bipolar disorder, are generally advised against using Ayahuasca. The powerful hallucinogenic effects of Ayahuasca can exacerbate existing psychological vulnerabilities and may lead to distressing experiences.

2. Medication Interactions:

- Ayahuasca contains compounds that can interact with certain medications, including antidepressants and other psychiatric drugs. These interactions can lead to dangerous or unpredictable effects. It is crucial to consult with a healthcare professional if you are taking any medications before considering Ayahuasca.

3. Physical Health:

- People with certain physical health conditions, such as heart problems, liver issues, or a history of seizures, should exercise caution when considering Ayahuasca. The brew can have effects on the cardiovascular system, and the purgative effects can be physically demanding.

4. Substance Abuse History:

- Individuals with a history of substance abuse may be at risk for negative outcomes during Ayahuasca ceremonies. Ayahuasca should not be viewed as a "quick fix" for addiction, and its use should be carefully considered and guided by professionals if it is being explored as a treatment option.

5. Legal and Safety Concerns:

- The legal status of Ayahuasca varies from country to country, and participating in ceremonies in unregulated or unsafe settings can pose significant risks. It is essential to attend Ayahuasca ceremonies only in legal and reputable centers, with experienced facilitators who prioritize safety and well-being.

6. Emotional Vulnerability:

- Ayahuasca experiences can be emotionally intense, and individuals who are emotionally fragile or in a state of crisis should be cautious. It is essential to be in a stable and supportive environment with skilled facilitators.

7. Integration and Preparation:

- Insufficient preparation and integration can lead to challenging or unsettling experiences. Adequate preparation, which includes understanding the process and setting intentions, and proper integration afterward, are crucial for maximizing the potential benefits and minimizing risks. It is imperative not to underestimate the importance of adhering to the preparation guidelines. These guidelines are designed to cleanse and prepare your body, making it easier for the plant medicine to work effectively and ensuring a smoother ceremonial process.

8. Respect for the Medicine:

- Ayahuasca is a sacred plant medicine and should be treated with the utmost respect. Approaching it with reverence and humility is essential for a meaningful and safe experience. Embracing the Spirit of the plant as both a Guide and Teacher, and approaching it with trust and respect, paves the way for deep healing. With the belief that the plant consistently acts in their best interest, providing the precise healing needed, one can more readily surrender and release. The Spirit of the plant stands as a beacon, guiding individuals toward enlightenment and liberation.

9. Set and Setting:

- The environment in which you participate in an Ayahuasca ceremony is of great importance. It should be tranquil, supportive, and conducive to introspection. Setting the right intention for your journey can influence the experience. The most important is that the surrounding must make one feel safe so the individual can relax, and let the healing take place.

10. Support System:

- It is advisable to have a strong support system, including experienced facilitators and trusted individuals who can provide emotional support during and after the Ayahuasca experience.

In summary, while Ayahuasca has the potential for therapeutic and transformative experiences, it is not without risks, and its use should be approached with care and caution. It is essential to consult with healthcare professionals, experienced practitioners, and reputable Ayahuasca centers when considering its use. Ensuring that you are in good physical and mental health, adhering to safety guidelines, and being well-informed are all critical steps to minimize risks and maximize the potential benefits of Ayahuasca.

- **The importance of a safe and supportive setting.**

The importance of a safe and supportive setting for Ayahuasca ceremonies cannot be overstated. It plays a pivotal role in the overall experience, well-being, and potential therapeutic benefits. Here's why a safe and supportive setting is crucial when working with Ayahuasca:

1. Emotional Safety:

- Ayahuasca can bring up deep emotions and unresolved issues. A safe setting, guided by experienced facilitators, provides emotional support and guidance to help individuals navigate these intense and often challenging emotional experiences. This support can be instrumental in preventing psychological distress.

2. Physical Safety:

- Ayahuasca can have purgative effects, leading to vomiting and diarrhea. A safe setting ensures that participants have access to clean facilities and assistance if needed. Additionally, a serene and well-maintained environment minimizes physical hazards.

3. Experienced Facilitators:

- Skilled and experienced facilitators or shamans play a critical role in ensuring the safety and effectiveness of Ayahuasca ceremonies. They guide the process, offer reassurance, and provide expert insight into the experience. Facilitators can help participants integrate their experiences and navigate challenging moments.

4. Set and Setting:

- The ambiance and energy of the ceremonial space are essential. A supportive environment, often with traditional elements and rituals, contributes to a sense of sacredness and safety. The set and setting are carefully designed to facilitate introspection and connection with the medicine.

5. Monitoring and Supervision:

- During the ceremony, facilitators closely monitor participants' well-being and responses to the medicine. If someone experiences distress, they can provide appropriate support or intervene when necessary.

6. Integration Support:

- A safe and supportive setting includes a structure for post-ceremony integration. This phase is crucial for making sense of the experience, understanding its significance, and applying the insights to one's daily life. Facilitators and support networks can help individuals in this integration process.

7. Peer Support:

- Sharing the Ayahuasca experience with others in a group setting can create a sense of community and camaraderie. Participants often find comfort and understanding in the presence of others who are on a similar journey.

8. Minimizing External Distractions:

- A safe and supportive environment minimizes external distractions, allowing participants to focus entirely on their inner experience. This enhances the depth and introspective quality of the journey.

9. Legal and Ethical Considerations:

- A legal and ethical setting ensures that participants are engaging in ceremonies that comply with local regulations and are conducted in an ethically responsible manner.

In summary, a safe and supportive setting for Ayahuasca ceremonies is essential for the physical, emotional, and psychological well-being of participants. It provides guidance, care, and a structured framework to ensure that the experience is positive, meaningful, and transformative. When considering Ayahuasca, individuals should prioritize participating in ceremonies with experienced and reputable facilitators, taking care to choose settings that prioritize safety and well-being.

- **The role of Ayahuasca in indigenous Amazonian spirituality.**

Ayahuasca plays a central and sacred role in the spirituality of many indigenous Amazonian cultures. It is often considered a powerful and revered plant teacher that connects individuals to the spiritual realms, fosters healing, and imparts wisdom. Here's an overview of the role of Ayahuasca in indigenous Amazonian spirituality:

1. Connection to the Spirit World:

- Ayahuasca is believed to be a conduit to the spirit world and is used by shamans and healers to establish contact with ancestral spirits, deities, and plant spirits. It is considered a gateway for communication with these entities, which provide guidance, knowledge, and healing.

2. Healing and Purification:

- Ayahuasca is viewed as a potent healer in indigenous Amazonian spirituality. It is used to address physical and spiritual ailments, cleanse the body and mind, and restore balance to the individual. The purgative effects of Ayahuasca are seen as a form of purifying the body and soul.

3. Visionary Insights:

- Ayahuasca ceremonies often involve the experience of vivid and profound visions. These visions are interpreted as messages from the spirit world, offering guidance and insights into one's life, purpose, and the nature of reality. They may also reveal the causes of physical or emotional ailments.

4. Plant Wisdom:

- Indigenous people in the Amazon rainforest have a deep connection with the plant world. Ayahuasca is considered a source of plant wisdom and knowledge, which can be used for both physical and spiritual healing. This wisdom includes the properties and uses of other medicinal plants.

5. Community and Traditions:

- Ayahuasca ceremonies are communal and sacred events in many indigenous cultures. They are often passed down through generations and are a fundamental part of community life. The rituals, songs, and prayers associated with Ayahuasca ceremonies are essential to preserving cultural and spiritual traditions.

6. Rites of Passage:

- Ayahuasca is used in various rites of passage, such as initiation ceremonies, where individuals receive spiritual guidance and blessings to mark significant life transitions. It is also used in rituals related to birth, marriage, and death.

7. Ecological Awareness:

- Indigenous cultures in the Amazon have a deep ecological awareness, and Ayahuasca is considered a tool for understanding and protecting the rainforest. It reinforces the belief that humans are an integral part of nature and emphasizes the importance of conserving the environment.

8. Ethical and Cultural Values:

- The use of Ayahuasca is often grounded in a set of ethical and cultural values. It reinforces the importance of reciprocity with nature, community support, and the preservation of indigenous knowledge and traditions.

It's important to recognize that Ayahuasca holds a different cultural and spiritual significance within indigenous Amazonian communities than it does in the context of Western or neo-shamanic practices. The indigenous use of Ayahuasca is deeply rooted in a complex and holistic worldview that encompasses nature, community, and the spiritual realms. It is considered a sacred and integral part of their way of life, offering a deep understanding of the interconnectedness of all things and a means to promote harmony within themselves and the natural world.

- **Its use as a tool for self-discovery and personal growth.**

Ayahuasca is increasingly recognized as a tool for self-discovery and personal growth in the context of Western and modern spiritual practices. While its traditional use in indigenous Amazonian cultures is deeply rooted in a different set of beliefs and rituals, in this context, Ayahuasca is often seen as a means for individuals to explore their inner selves, gain insight, and foster personal growth. Here are some ways in which Ayahuasca can be used for self-discovery and personal development:

1. Deep Self-Exploration:

- Ayahuasca journeys can lead individuals to explore their inner landscapes, uncovering hidden thoughts, emotions, and memories. It allows for a deep examination of one's psyche, often leading to a better understanding of oneself.

2. Healing and Catharsis:

- Ayahuasca can facilitate the release of repressed emotions, trauma, and unresolved issues. This emotional catharsis can lead to healing and a sense of emotional relief, enabling personal growth and transformation.

3. Insight and Clarity:

- Ayahuasca often provides profound insights and clarity about one's life, relationships, and personal challenges. These insights can inspire positive changes and lead to a greater sense of purpose and direction.

4. Integration of Experiences:

- The integration of Ayahuasca experiences is a vital part of the personal growth process. This phase involves reflecting on the insights gained during the ceremony and finding ways to apply them to everyday life. Integration can lead to lasting positive changes.

5. Confronting Fears and Limiting Beliefs:

- Ayahuasca may help individuals confront deep-seated fears, limiting beliefs, and negative thought patterns. By facing and working through these obstacles, people often experience personal growth and increased self-confidence.

6. Increased Mindfulness and Awareness:

- Ayahuasca can heighten awareness of one's thoughts, emotions, and behaviors, fostering greater mindfulness. This increased awareness can lead to more conscious and intentional decision-making.

7. Enhanced Creativity and Problem Solving:

- Many individuals report increased creativity and improved problem-solving abilities following Ayahuasca experiences. It can help break through creative blocks and inspire new ideas and perspectives.

8. Strengthening Spirituality:

- Ayahuasca experiences often lead to a deepened sense of spirituality, connection to the universe, and a greater understanding of the self in a broader context. This can be a source of personal growth and enrichment.

9. Emotional Resilience:

- The emotional challenges that can arise during Ayahuasca journeys, including confronting difficult emotions and fears, can build emotional resilience and coping skills. This personal growth often results in greater emotional balance.

It's important to emphasize that Ayahuasca is a powerful and potentially challenging tool for personal growth. The experiences can vary widely, and they are best undertaken in a safe and supportive environment with experienced facilitators. Participants should approach Ayahuasca with a respectful and responsible mindset, keeping in mind that personal growth often involves confronting and working through difficult emotions and experiences. The integration of these experiences into everyday life is crucial for lasting personal growth and positive transformation.

Ayahuasca Ceremonies
- **An overview of traditional Ayahuasca ceremonies.**

Traditional Ayahuasca ceremonies are sacred and ritualistic events conducted by indigenous Amazonian communities. These ceremonies have been practiced for centuries and hold a profound cultural and spiritual significance. Here is an overview of the key elements and practices of traditional Ayahuasca ceremonies:

1. Preparation and Intention Setting:

- Ayahuasca ceremonies begin with a period of preparation. This may involve dietary restrictions, abstinence from certain substances, and specific rituals to purify the body and mind. Participants are encouraged to set clear intentions for their journey, which may include seeking healing, insights, or spiritual guidance.

2. Ceremonial Space:

- The ceremony takes place in a carefully prepared, sacred space. This space is often adorned with natural elements, such as leaves, flowers, and candles, and is considered a spiritual portal. It is designed to create a safe, harmonious, and focused environment for the ceremony.

3. Shaman or Healer Guidance:

- An experienced shaman or healer, often referred to as an "ayahuasquero" or "curandero," leads the ceremony. The shaman is seen as a spiritual guide, capable of connecting with the spirit world and facilitating healing and insights. They are responsible for the safety and well-being of participants.

4. Ayahuasca Brew:

- The Ayahuasca brew is prepared by the shaman or healer using the Banisteriopsis caapi vine and the leaves of the Psychotria viridis shrub. These plants contain the psychoactive compounds necessary for the ceremony. The brew is often blessed, and the shaman may sing icaros (healing songs) to infuse it with spiritual power.

5. Ingesting Ayahuasca:

- Participants typically ingest the Ayahuasca brew after a series of blessings, prayers, and ceremonial rituals. It is common for participants to drink the brew one by one. The shaman may also drink Ayahuasca and chant icaros to guide the participants' journeys.

6. Music and Chants:

- Throughout the ceremony, the shaman and other participants may sing sacred songs or chants called icaros. These melodies are believed to have healing and protective qualities and help guide the experience. The music is a fundamental element of the ceremony.

7. Visions and Insights:

- Ayahuasca typically induces powerful visions and altered states of consciousness. Participants may experience a range of visual, emotional, and spiritual insights. These visions and experiences are interpreted as messages from the spirit world, providing guidance and healing.

8. Healing and Purging:

- Many Ayahuasca ceremonies involve purging, which can include vomiting and, less commonly, diarrhea. This is often considered a form of cleansing, purifying both the body and the spirit. It is referred to as "the purge."

9. Integration and Sharing:

- After the Ayahuasca experience, participants often gather to share their experiences and insights. This phase is essential for integration, allowing individuals to make sense of their journey and apply the lessons learned to their lives.

10. Respect for Nature:

- Ayahuasca ceremonies often emphasize the interconnectedness of all life forms and the importance of protecting the environment. Participants are encouraged to respect and preserve the natural world.

Traditional Ayahuasca ceremonies are deeply rooted in indigenous cosmology and cultural practices. They are considered a form of traditional medicine and spiritual communion. Participants are expected to approach these ceremonies with reverence, humility, and a commitment to cultural respect and sustainability. While Ayahuasca ceremonies are now practiced in various parts of the world, it is important to remember that the traditional context holds a unique and profound significance within indigenous Amazonian cultures.

- **The importance of trained shamans or facilitators.**

The presence of trained shamans or experienced facilitators in Ayahuasca ceremonies is of paramount importance for several crucial reasons. These knowledgeable guides play a central role in ensuring the safety, effectiveness, and ethical conduct of the ceremonies. Here's why trained shamans or facilitators are so vital:

1. Safety and Well-Being:

- Experienced shamans and facilitators have a deep understanding of Ayahuasca and its effects. They are well-equipped to monitor participants during the ceremony, respond to any physical or emotional distress, and ensure the overall safety and well-being of those involved.

2. Expertise in Plant Medicine:

- Shamans and facilitators are often well-versed in the properties and uses of various medicinal plants in addition to Ayahuasca. This knowledge is instrumental in creating the Ayahuasca brew and may involve adding other plants to address specific health issues or enhance the ceremonial experience.

3. Guidance and Support:

- Trained shamans and facilitators are skilled at guiding participants through the journey. They can offer reassurance, insight, and spiritual guidance during moments of confusion or emotional intensity. This guidance can be vital for individuals to navigate the Ayahuasca experience.

4. Ethical Conduct:

- Experienced facilitators uphold ethical standards in conducting ceremonies. They respect the sacredness of the Ayahuasca brew, follow cultural and spiritual protocols, and ensure that participants are treated with dignity and respect. This helps maintain the integrity of the ceremony.

5. Cultural Context:

- Trained shamans are often deeply rooted in indigenous Amazonian culture and cosmology. They can provide cultural context and traditional elements that enhance the ceremony's significance and authenticity. This enriches the spiritual experience and deepens participants' understanding of Ayahuasca.

6. Legal and Safety Compliance:

- Experienced facilitators are often well-versed in local and international legal requirements for Ayahuasca ceremonies. This knowledge ensures that the ceremonies are conducted in compliance with regulations and prioritize safety.

7. Integration and Post-Ceremony Support:

- Shamans and facilitators are valuable in the post-ceremony phase, helping participants integrate their experiences into their daily lives. They provide a framework for understanding the insights gained and offer guidance on how to apply them for personal growth.

8. Cultural Preservation:

- Trained shamans play a role in preserving indigenous cultural traditions and protecting the knowledge and wisdom associated with Ayahuasca. Supporting these practitioners contributes to the preservation of cultural heritage.

9. Community and Peer Support:

- The presence of a shaman or facilitator fosters a sense of community and peer support among participants. This shared experience can create a supportive and understanding environment that enhances the journey.

10. Responsiveness to Individual Needs:

- Experienced facilitators are sensitive to the unique needs of each participant. They can tailor the ceremony to address specific intentions, challenges, or goals, allowing for a more personalized and transformative experience.

In summary, trained shamans or facilitators are essential for creating a safe, culturally respectful, and spiritually significant Ayahuasca experience. They bring expertise, guidance, and an understanding of the ceremonial process that is invaluable for those seeking the benefits of Ayahuasca in a responsible and transformative manner. When considering an Ayahuasca ceremony, individuals should prioritize participating in those led by experienced and reputable facilitators who adhere to ethical, safety, and cultural standards if you choose to heal by yourself and take it alone in your home like westerners have been doing recently especially in Europe and USA then make sure the shaman who provided you with the medicine have guided you with all the instructions, icaros or healing chants and songs in a playlist form, all the preparation regarding foods before and after the ceremony is included and that he is available in case you have questions or need special informations before or after your ceremonies. .

Legal Status of Ayahuasca
- **The legal framework around Ayahuasca in different countries.**

The legal status of Ayahuasca varies from country to country, and it is subject to a complex and evolving legal landscape. In many places, Ayahuasca exists in a legal gray area due to its unique status as a plant-based entheogen used for spiritual, religious, and therapeutic purposes. The legal framework can change over time, so it's essential to stay informed about the specific regulations in your country. Here is a general overview of the legal status of Ayahuasca in different countries:

1. Peru:

- Peru is known for its long history of Ayahuasca use and has established legal protections for its traditional and cultural use by indigenous communities. The country recognizes Ayahuasca as part of its cultural heritage. It is legal for traditional and spiritual use, provided it is conducted by trained shamans.

2. Brazil:

- In Brazil, Ayahuasca is legal for religious use within specific religious organizations, such as the Santo Daime and the União do Vegetal (UDV). The use of Ayahuasca in these contexts has been recognized as a constitutional right.

3. Colombia:

- Colombia's legal status regarding Ayahuasca is complex. In 2010, the Colombian Constitutional Court decriminalized the use of Ayahuasca for spiritual and religious purposes, but the specifics of regulation and enforcement can vary by region.

4. United States:

- Ayahuasca is classified as a Schedule I controlled substance in the United States, which means it is illegal for recreational use. However, some religious organizations, such as the Santo Daime and the UDV, have successfully argued for exemptions under the Religious Freedom Restoration Act, allowing them to use Ayahuasca legally in their religious practices.

5. Canada:

- Canada's legal framework for Ayahuasca is similar to that of the United States. It is considered a controlled substance, and its use is illegal for recreational purposes. However, the courts have granted exemptions to religious organizations, allowing them to use Ayahuasca as part of their spiritual practices.

6. European Union:

- Ayahuasca's legal status in European countries can vary widely. Some countries, such as Spain and Portugal, have relatively permissive approaches and allow Ayahuasca ceremonies. In contrast, other countries, like France and the UK, have stricter regulations.

7. Australia:

- Australia has a complex legal framework, and the legality of Ayahuasca can vary between states and territories. Some areas have implemented strict regulations, while others have taken a more permissive stance, allowing Ayahuasca use within certain contexts.

8. Other Countries:

- The legal status of Ayahuasca in many countries can be uncertain, as it often falls into a gray area. In some places, it may be tolerated for personal or spiritual use, while in others, it may be subject to legal restrictions.

It's crucial to understand the legal regulations and cultural context of Ayahuasca in your specific location. Always ensure that any ceremonies you attend are conducted within the boundaries of local laws and in a responsible, safe, and respectful manner. The legal status of Ayahuasca can change over time due to evolving perspectives and policies, so it's essential to stay informed and seek legal guidance if needed.

How to Prepare for an Ayahuasca Experience
- **Guidelines for individuals considering an Ayahuasca journey.**

Preparing for an Ayahuasca experience is a critical step to ensure a safe, meaningful, and transformative journey. Here are some guidelines for individuals considering an Ayahuasca ceremony:

1. Research and Education:

- Start by researching Ayahuasca, its effects, and its cultural and spiritual significance. Understand the potential risks and benefits associated with Ayahuasca. Reading books, articles, and seeking information from reputable sources can help you make an informed decision.

2. Choose a Reputable Ayahuasca Center:

- If you decide to proceed, choose a reputable and legal Ayahuasca center or retreat. Research the center's background, facilitators, and reviews. Ensure that they operate in compliance with local regulations and prioritize safety and ethical conduct.

3. Consult with a Healthcare Professional:

- If you have any pre-existing medical conditions, are taking medications, or have specific health concerns, consult with a healthcare professional. Ayahuasca can interact with certain medications and may not be suitable for everyone.

4. Set Clear Intentions:

- Reflect on your reasons for wanting to experience Ayahuasca and set clear intentions for your journey. This can help guide your experience and personal growth.

5. Diet and Abstinence:

- Many Ayahuasca centers recommend following a specific diet in the days leading up to the ceremony. This typically involves avoiding certain foods, alcohol, and other substances. The purpose is to prepare your body and mind for the experience and reduce the risk of adverse reactions.

6. Physical and Mental Preparation:

- Engage in practices that support your physical and mental well-being. This may include regular exercise, meditation, yoga, or other mindfulness techniques. Prepare your body and mind to be in the best possible state.

7. Set and Setting:

- Choose a supportive and peaceful environment for your ceremony. The setting should be comfortable, safe, and conducive to introspection. Create a space that promotes a sense of tranquility and reverence.

8. Ceremony Etiquette:

- Familiarize yourself with the etiquette and protocols of Ayahuasca ceremonies. Be respectful of the shaman, facilitators, and fellow participants. Follow the guidance provided during the ceremony.

9. Be Open and Surrender:

- Approach the Ayahuasca experience with an open mind and a willingness to surrender to the process. Let go of expectations and allow the medicine to guide you. Resistance can lead to a more challenging experience.

10. Support System:

- Inform a trusted friend or family member about your Ayahuasca journey, including the location and contact details of the retreat center. Having a support system in place can provide comfort and assistance if needed.

11. Aftercare and Integration:

- Plan for post-ceremony integration. Understand that the insights gained during the experience may require reflection and integration into your daily life. Many Ayahuasca centers offer integration support or provide resources to help you make sense of your journey.

12. Legal and Ethical Considerations:

- Ensure that the Ayahuasca ceremony you are attending complies with local regulations and ethical standards. Be aware of the legal status of Ayahuasca in your country and the location of the ceremony.

Remember that Ayahuasca is a powerful and potentially intense experience. By following these guidelines and preparing thoroughly, you can maximize the benefits of your Ayahuasca journey and ensure a safe and meaningful experience. Approach Ayahuasca with respect, reverence, and a commitment to self-discovery and personal growth.

- **Dietary restrictions and mental preparation.**

Dietary restrictions and mental preparation are crucial aspects of preparing for an Ayahuasca experience. These practices help create a safe and conducive environment for the ceremony and allow you to get the most out of your journey. Here's a closer look at each of these elements:

Dietary Restrictions:

Avoid Certain Foods:
- In the days leading up to your Ayahuasca ceremony, it is typically recommended to avoid certain foods that may interact negatively with Ayahuasca or create discomfort during the experience. Common restrictions include:
    - Alcohol: Refrain from consuming alcohol, as it can have adverse interactions with Ayahuasca.
    - Caffeine: Limit or eliminate caffeine intake, as it may affect your ability to relax during the ceremony.
    - Spices and Salt: Avoid spicy, salty, and heavily seasoned foods, as they can irritate the stomach and digestive system.
    - Processed and Heavy Foods: Opt for light, simple, and easily digestible foods. Processed and heavy meals can lead to discomfort or nausea during the ceremony.
    - Pork and Red Meat: In some traditions, it is recommended to abstain from pork and red meat.

Consume Clean, Plant-Based Foods:
- Focus on a diet that consists of clean, plant-based, and easily digestible foods. This may include fresh fruits, vegetables, grains, legumes, and herbal teas. Eating lightly can help you feel more in tune with your body and facilitate the Ayahuasca experience.

Stay Hydrated:
- Drink plenty of water and herbal teas in the days leading up to the ceremony to stay well-hydrated.

Mental Preparation:

Set Clear Intentions:
- Spend time reflecting on your intentions for the Ayahuasca experience. What do you hope to gain from it? Setting clear intentions can guide your journey and help you focus on your personal growth goals.

Mindfulness and Meditation:
- Engage in mindfulness and meditation practices to cultivate self-awareness and mental clarity. These practices can help you stay present during the ceremony.

Release Expectations:
- Let go of preconceived notions and expectations about what the Ayahuasca experience should be like. Each journey is unique, and surrendering to the process is essential for a meaningful experience.

Emotional Preparedness:

- Be prepared to confront and work through challenging emotions or past traumas that may surface during the ceremony. A willingness to explore these aspects of yourself is a key part of personal growth.

Embrace Surrender:

- Understand that Ayahuasca is a powerful teacher. Surrender to the process and trust in the wisdom of the medicine. Resistance can lead to more challenging experiences.

Emphasize Self-Care:

- Prioritize self-care in the days leading up to the ceremony. Engage in practices that promote relaxation and self-compassion.

Journaling:

- Consider keeping a journal to record your thoughts, emotions, and reflections as you prepare for the ceremony. Journaling can be a valuable tool for personal growth and self-discovery.

Speak with a Counselor or Therapist:

- If you have unresolved emotional issues or trauma, consider seeking support from a therapist or counselor. Discussing your concerns with a mental health professional can help you prepare for the Ayahuasca experience.

By following these dietary restrictions and engaging in effective mental preparation, you can optimize your readiness for an Ayahuasca journey. These practices help create a supportive and harmonious environment for the ceremony, allowing you to approach the experience with mindfulness, intention, and a commitment to personal growth and self-discovery.

Ayahuasca and Modern Research

- **Recent scientific studies and clinical trials.**

Ayahuasca has gained significant attention from the scientific and medical communities in recent years. While research on Ayahuasca is still in its early stages, a growing body of studies and clinical trials has explored its potential therapeutic benefits and mechanisms of action. Here are some recent scientific studies and clinical trials related to Ayahuasca:

1. Ayahuasca and Depression:

- Several studies have investigated the potential of Ayahuasca as a treatment for depression. Research suggests that the brew may have fast-acting antidepressant effects. Clinical trials have explored its impact on mood and depressive symptoms.

2. Ayahuasca and Anxiety Disorders:

- Some studies have examined Ayahuasca's effects on anxiety disorders, such as generalized anxiety disorder and social anxiety. Preliminary findings suggest that Ayahuasca may reduce anxiety and improve overall well-being.

3. Ayahuasca and PTSD:

- Clinical trials have been initiated to investigate Ayahuasca's potential in the treatment of post-traumatic stress disorder (PTSD). Early research suggests that Ayahuasca may help individuals process traumatic experiences and reduce PTSD symptoms.

4. Ayahuasca and Substance Use Disorders:

- Research has explored Ayahuasca's potential in treating substance use disorders, including alcohol and drug addiction. Some studies indicate that Ayahuasca may promote abstinence and reduce cravings.

5. Ayahuasca and Neuroplasticity:

- Studies have examined the impact of Ayahuasca on brain function and neuroplasticity. Research suggests that Ayahuasca may enhance neural connectivity and promote structural changes in the brain.

6. Ayahuasca and Mindfulness:

- Some research has explored the link between Ayahuasca experiences and enhanced mindfulness and psychological well-being. Ayahuasca ceremonies have been associated with increased mindfulness and introspection.

7. Mechanisms of Action:

- Research has delved into the pharmacological and neurobiological mechanisms of Ayahuasca. Studies have looked at the role of the active compounds, such as DMT and harmine, and how they affect neurotransmitter systems and brain function.

8. Safety and Adverse Effects:

- Clinical trials and studies have assessed the safety and potential adverse effects of Ayahuasca. Researchers have investigated the physiological and psychological risks associated with its use.

9. Legal and Ethical Considerations:

- Research has also addressed the legal and ethical aspects of Ayahuasca use in clinical and therapeutic settings. Studies examine the regulation and ethical conduct of Ayahuasca-assisted therapy.

It's important to note that while these studies and trials provide promising insights, Ayahuasca is a powerful and complex substance, and its use must be approached with caution and responsibility. Clinical research is ongoing, and further studies are needed to establish the safety and efficacy of Ayahuasca for specific therapeutic applications. Additionally, it is essential to participate in Ayahuasca-related research and therapeutic interventions within legal and ethical frameworks.

- **The potential future of Ayahuasca in mainstream medicine.**

The potential future of Ayahuasca in mainstream medicine is a topic of growing interest and exploration. While there are many challenges and questions to address, several factors suggest that Ayahuasca could play a role in mainstream medicine in the future:

1. Clinical Research: Ongoing clinical research is exploring Ayahuasca's potential therapeutic benefits, particularly in the treatment of mental health conditions like depression, anxiety, and PTSD. As more rigorous scientific studies are conducted, the evidence supporting the efficacy and safety of Ayahuasca-assisted therapy may continue to accumulate.

2. Fast-Acting Antidepressant: Ayahuasca has shown promise as a fast-acting antidepressant in some studies. This could be particularly significant in addressing the limitations of current antidepressant medications, which often take weeks to produce noticeable effects.

3. Addressing Treatment-Resistant Conditions: Ayahuasca has demonstrated potential in treating conditions that are often resistant to conventional treatments,

such as treatment-resistant depression and PTSD. This could open up new possibilities for individuals who have not responded to traditional therapies.

4. Integration with Psychotherapy: Ayahuasca-assisted psychotherapy involves a structured and therapeutic context, integrating the use of Ayahuasca with psychological support. This model aligns with the principles of evidence-based psychotherapy, making it potentially more palatable to mainstream medical practices.

5. Mental Health Crisis: The increasing prevalence of mental health disorders has created a sense of urgency to explore new treatment options. Ayahuasca may offer an alternative approach that addresses the root causes of psychological distress, rather than merely managing symptoms.

6. Ethical and Legal Frameworks: As research progresses, the development of ethical and legal frameworks for the use of Ayahuasca in clinical settings becomes essential. Regulating its use to ensure safety and patient well-being is an important step toward mainstream acceptance.

7. Cultural and Spiritual Respect: Ayahuasca's spiritual and cultural significance is recognized and respected. Integrating these aspects into therapeutic practices may enhance the effectiveness of Ayahuasca-assisted therapy and promote a more holistic approach to healing.

8. Public Interest and Demand: There is a growing public interest in alternative and complementary treatments for mental health and well-being. As more individuals seek Ayahuasca therapy, mainstream medicine may respond to meet this demand.

9. Collaboration and Training: Collaboration between traditional Ayahuasca practitioners, medical professionals, and therapists can provide a bridge between indigenous wisdom and modern clinical practices. Training programs are emerging to ensure that facilitators are well-prepared and responsible.

10. Evidence-Based Medicine: Mainstream medicine is increasingly embracing evidence-based approaches. As the scientific evidence supporting Ayahuasca's therapeutic potential continues to develop, it may gain acceptance within the medical community.

While the future of Ayahuasca in mainstream medicine is promising, it also raises important questions about safety, regulation, ethics, and cultural respect. Collaboration, research, and responsible practices will be essential as Ayahuasca moves toward potential integration into mainstream healthcare. As this journey continues, it will be crucial to strike a balance between the preservation of indigenous traditions and the responsible, evidence-based use of Ayahuasca for the benefit of individuals seeking healing and personal growth.

Conclusion
- **A summary of key points.**

In conclusion, Ayahuasca is a complex and fascinating plant medicine with a rich history and a promising future. Here's a more detailed summary of the key points covered in this discussion:

Ayahuasca's Essence:
- Ayahuasca is a psychoactive brew made from the Banisteriopsis caapi vine and the leaves of the Psychotria viridis shrub. It is revered for its deep-rooted spiritual, healing, and shamanic significance in indigenous Amazonian cultures.

Historical and Cultural Significance:
- Ayahuasca use dates back centuries among indigenous Amazonian communities. It has been integral to their cultural and spiritual practices, serving as a means of connecting with the spirit world, receiving guidance, and promoting healing.

The Ayahuasca Experience:
- Ayahuasca journeys are profound and transformative. They involve altered states of consciousness, vivid visions, deep introspection, and often physical purging. These experiences are seen as a form of cleansing, healing, and revelation.

Health Benefits and Therapeutic Potential:
- Ayahuasca is increasingly being explored for its potential therapeutic benefits. Research suggests it may have a role in treating various mental health conditions, including depression, anxiety, post-traumatic stress disorder (PTSD), and substance use disorders.

Research and Mental Health:
- Scientific studies and clinical trials are actively investigating Ayahuasca's effectiveness in treating mental health issues. Promising results suggest it could offer fast-acting relief and long-term healing for individuals who have not responded to conventional treatments.

Risks and Precautions:

- Ayahuasca is not without risks, and it's crucial for individuals to understand potential contraindications and safety measures. Psychological and physical preparation are necessary to ensure a safe and beneficial experience.

The Importance of a Supportive Setting:

- The presence of trained shamans or experienced facilitators is critical for providing guidance, safety, and cultural context during Ayahuasca ceremonies. A safe and supportive environment is essential for participants to navigate the intense journey.

Indigenous Spirituality and Wisdom:

- Ayahuasca is deeply ingrained in indigenous Amazonian spirituality and cosmology. It plays a central role in their belief systems and serves as a means of connecting with the divine and gaining wisdom.

Self-Discovery and Personal Growth:

- Many individuals use Ayahuasca as a tool for deep self-exploration, healing, and personal growth. It can help individuals confront fears, limiting beliefs, and unresolved emotions while fostering mindfulness and increased self-awareness.

Ayahuasca Ceremonies:

- Traditional Ayahuasca ceremonies are sacred rituals led by experienced shamans. They involve careful preparation, intention setting, and the consumption of Ayahuasca in a ceremonial context, with music and chanting.

Trained Shamans and Facilitators:

- Experienced shamans and facilitators are central to ensuring the safety, cultural respect, and therapeutic potential of Ayahuasca ceremonies. Their expertise and guidance are essential for a positive experience.

Legal Status Worldwide:

- The legal status of Ayahuasca varies from country to country, often existing in a legal gray area due to its unique cultural and spiritual significance. Some nations recognize its value in traditional practices, while others maintain strict regulations.

Future in Mainstream Medicine:

- Ayahuasca's potential integration into mainstream medicine is a topic of increasing interest. As clinical research continues, public curiosity grows, and the need for novel treatments for mental health conditions persists, Ayahuasca may find a place within conventional healthcare practices.

The future of Ayahuasca is marked by a delicate balance between respecting indigenous traditions and responsibly integrating this powerful plant medicine into modern society. As interest and research continue to evolve, it is essential to maintain a focus on ethical, safe, and evidence-based use to ensure the well-being and personal growth of individuals seeking healing and transformation.

- **Encouraging responsible and informed use of Ayahuasca.**

Encouraging responsible and informed use of Ayahuasca is paramount to ensure the well-being and safety of individuals who embark on this profound journey. Here are key steps to promote responsible and informed Ayahuasca use:

1. Education and Research:

- Promote education about Ayahuasca, its history, cultural significance, and potential effects. Encourage individuals to research reputable sources and gain a deep understanding of what they are undertaking.

2. Seek Legal and Ethical Frameworks:

- Emphasize the importance of participating in Ayahuasca ceremonies that operate within legal and ethical frameworks. This includes seeking ceremonies held by experienced facilitators and shamans who prioritize safety and cultural respect.

3. Medical Assessment:

- Advise individuals to undergo a medical assessment before engaging in an Ayahuasca ceremony, especially if they have pre-existing medical conditions or are taking medications. A healthcare professional can help determine their suitability.

4. Set Clear Intentions:

- Encourage participants to set clear and meaningful intentions for their Ayahuasca journey. This can guide the experience and provide a focus for personal growth and healing.

5. Preparation and Integration:

- Stress the importance of both physical and mental preparation. Engage in mindfulness practices, meditation, and introspection before the ceremony. Also, highlight the significance of post-ceremony integration to make sense of the insights gained.

6. Responsible Ceremony Selection:

- Advise individuals to select Ayahuasca ceremonies carefully. Research the background of the retreat center or shaman, read reviews, and ensure the ceremony adheres to safety and ethical standards.

7. Trust the Process:

- Encourage participants to approach Ayahuasca with an open mind and surrender to the process. Resistance can lead to a more challenging experience, so emphasize the importance of trust and letting go.

8. Respect the Medicine:

- Instill a deep respect for Ayahuasca as a powerful teacher and healer. Encourage individuals to approach it with reverence and humility, recognizing its potential to offer profound insights.
- Deep respect for the shamans, facilitators and those who have sourced you with the medicine is very important, and it's always recommended to support the tribes and the places where the medicine comes from. This is a significant way to show respect and gratitude for the medicine and its origin. To help to look after the amazon rainforest and the people who are keepers of the forest is one of the teachings of ayahuasca.

9. Support System:

- Stress the importance of informing a trusted friend or family member about the Ayahuasca journey. Having a support system in place can provide emotional comfort and assistance if needed.

10. Cultural Awareness: - Foster an understanding of the cultural and spiritual significance of Ayahuasca in indigenous Amazonian communities. Encourage individuals to approach the medicine with respect for its origins.

11. Promote Ethical and Legal Considerations: - Advocate for the responsible and legal use of Ayahuasca, respecting the local laws and regulations in place. This ensures a safe and respectful approach to this sacred tradition.

12. Ongoing Education: - Encourage individuals to continue learning and seeking knowledge about Ayahuasca even after their journey. This can help them make sense of their experiences and integrate the insights into their lives.

13. Share Personal Experiences Responsibly: - If individuals choose to share their Ayahuasca experiences with others, emphasize the importance of doing so responsibly and without sensationalism. This can help demystify Ayahuasca while conveying its potential benefits and challenges.

Promoting responsible and informed use of Ayahuasca is not only essential for personal safety but also for the preservation of the cultural and spiritual significance of this ancient tradition. By approaching Ayahuasca with reverence, awareness, and mindfulness, individuals can harness its potential for healing, personal growth, and transformation in a responsible and informed manner.

- **Recent scientific studies and clinical trials.**

In recent years, scientific interest in Ayahuasca has surged, with numerous studies and clinical trials exploring its potential therapeutic effects. While my last knowledge update was in September 2023, there have likely been further developments in Ayahuasca research. Here's an overview of some noteworthy recent scientific studies and clinical trials:

Depression and Anxiety Studies: Researchers have conducted studies to investigate Ayahuasca's impact on depression and anxiety. Preliminary findings suggest that Ayahuasca may have the potential to alleviate symptoms and enhance overall well-being.

Addiction Treatment: Clinical trials have been initiated to assess Ayahuasca's efficacy in treating substance addictions, including alcohol and drug dependencies. Initial results indicate promise in aiding individuals with addiction issues.

Post-Traumatic Stress Disorder (PTSD): Some studies have explored Ayahuasca as a treatment for PTSD. Early research shows promise in reducing symptoms and improving the mental health of those affected by this condition.

Neurological and Cognitive Effects: Utilizing neuroimaging techniques, researchers have delved into the neurological effects of Ayahuasca. These investigations provide insights into the brain mechanisms involved in Ayahuasca experiences.

Spirituality and Belief Changes: Research has focused on Ayahuasca's impact on spirituality and personal beliefs. Some studies indicate that Ayahuasca experiences can lead to profound spiritual insights and shifts in worldview.

Psychotherapeutic Benefits: Clinical trials are underway to assess the potential of Ayahuasca-assisted psychotherapy for various mental health conditions. This approach combines Ayahuasca experiences with therapeutic sessions to maximize therapeutic benefits.

Long-Term Outcomes: Longitudinal studies have tracked participants over extended periods to assess the enduring effects of Ayahuasca experiences on mental health and overall well-being. This research helps understand the lasting impact of Ayahuasca use.

Additional Health Considerations: Beyond mental health, Ayahuasca has been investigated for its potential in addressing other health conditions, including chronic pain, cluster headaches, and even Parkinson's disease. These studies aim to expand our understanding of the diverse applications of Ayahuasca.

As Ayahuasca research continues to evolve, it holds the promise of offering valuable therapeutic insights and solutions across a range of conditions. To stay current with the latest developments in Ayahuasca research, it's advisable to consult academic databases, clinical trial registries, and websites of respected research institutions and organizations focused on psychedelic and plant medicine research.

- **The potential future of Ayahuasca in mainstream medicine.**

The potential future of Ayahuasca in mainstream medicine is nothing short of a promising revolution—a vibrant tapestry of healing, wisdom, and transformation woven into the very fabric of healthcare. As the mists of ancient Amazonian traditions continue to part, revealing the profound benefits of this sacred brew, the medical landscape stands poised for an exhilarating shift.

Picture a future where Ayahuasca, the queen of the rainforest, is welcomed into the hallowed halls of mainstream medicine. Where its mystical synergy of plant compounds and spiritual insights is not only acknowledged but celebrated as a powerful tool for healing.

In this visionary realm, Ayahuasca-assisted therapies are embraced as a cornerstone of holistic healthcare. They offer individuals struggling with mental health challenges, addiction, and trauma an alternative path toward recovery—one that transcends mere symptom management and dives deep into the roots of the soul.

Imagine Ayahuasca retreat centers becoming therapeutic sanctuaries, offering a safe space for profound transformation and self-discovery. A place where seasoned healers and medical professionals collaborate, seamlessly integrating ancient wisdom with modern science.

As science continues to unlock the biochemical mysteries of Ayahuasca, we may see a new generation of pharmacological innovations inspired by its intricate chemical composition. Novel treatments for conditions such as depression, anxiety, and addiction may emerge, influenced by the ancient brew's wisdom.

This future is one where cultural respect and ethical considerations are paramount, where indigenous communities are partners, not just observers. The guardians of these traditions are honored, and their knowledge is valued for its timeless relevance.

The potential future of Ayahuasca in mainstream medicine is a journey of hope and possibility, where the ancient and the modern dance in harmony, and where the human spirit is liberated to explore the uncharted realms of consciousness. It's a realm where healing, wisdom, and transformation converge in a symphony of well-being—a future that, like Ayahuasca itself, promises to be a source of profound renewal for the body, mind, and soul.

Bonus

- **Shamanic Empowerment with Ayahuasca Herself**

Keep your eyes half open and let your imagination carry you to the heart of the Amazon rainforest. The air is thick with the scents of lush foliage, and the vibrant hues of emerald leaves and exotic flowers paint the landscape in every shade imaginable. The symphony of the jungle fills your ears as you sit by a crackling bonfire, the flickering flames casting shadows that dance with the spirits of the forest.

An elder shaman, adorned in intricate patterns of vibrant colors, approaches you with a carved wooden cup filled with the sacred Ayahuasca brew. You accept the cup with reverence, feeling the ancient energy pulsating within it. As you drink, the world around you comes to life in a dazzling display of colors and sounds. The forest itself seems to exhale a deep, resonant hum, as if welcoming you into its very soul.

As the Ayahuasca takes hold, the forest embraces you in its nurturing arms. Ancient trees with gnarled bark reach out to bless you with their wisdom, offering you the strength and resilience of the ages. A vibrant macaw perches nearby, its feathers shimmering with every color of the rainbow. It gazes into your eyes and imparts the gift of vibrant expression, encouraging you to speak your truth.

A majestic jaguar prowls through the undergrowth, bestowing upon you the grace and power of the feline spirit. The jaguar's eyes hold the secrets of the night, and you feel the courage to explore the depths of your own shadow.

The night unfolds, and the shaman's icaros resonate through the forest, painting the colors of your visions. You are surrounded by a chorus of spirit animals and plant allies, each offering their blessings. The wise old Ceiba tree extends its branches, connecting you to the heavens and the earth. The playful river dolphin offers the gift of joy and playfulness, inviting you to dance with the currents of life.

As the journey deepens, a sense of purging arises. In the act of releasing, you witness all that held you back—fear, doubt, pain—leaving your being, never to return. With the purge comes an overwhelming relief, and your body feels light, cleansed, and pure.

The world becomes a tapestry of beauty, every leaf glistening with dew, every sound an exquisite melody. You delight in the connection to all things, and nature's secrets are laid bare before you.

And then, in the zenith of your journey, a spectacular moment unfolds. Ayahuasca herself emerges as a luminous white serpent adorned with radiant rainbow patterns. She approaches, entering your body through your heart and crown, and you feel a profound connection to the very spirit of Ayahuasca. She whispers, "From now on, I will protect you and keep you healthy, blessed, and safe during your awakening journey. I will drive away all negative spirits and emotions that approach you, and I will gift you with auspicious dreams."

As her blessing unfolds, the world transforms into a radiant pink hue, and rose petals gently rain down upon your head, symbolizing the purity and love that surrounds you.

The shaman's voice gently breaks the spell, "The session is over for today. You can now go to sleep." As you close your eyes to rest, the enchanting scenes of this vivid meditation leave you with a deep sense of gratitude, connection, and blissful serenity. You drift into a peaceful and rejuvenating sleep, feeling blessed and protected, embraced by the loving spirit of Ayahuasca and the rainforest.

Meet the 3 Elders keepers of sacred knowledge

Keep your eyes half open and let your imagination carry you to the magnificent mountains that resemble Cusco or Machu Picchu. As you stand amidst the towering peaks, the air is crisp, and the golden rays of the setting sun paint the landscape in warm hues of red and orange. You sense the magic of this sacred place.

In this mystical setting, you find yourself invited to join three revered elders, each carrying the supernatural shamanic wisdom of their respective cultures—the Incas, the Mayas, and the Aztecs. Together, you embark on a transformative journey under the starry night sky, gathered around a flickering bonfire, and the hypnotic beat of a shamanic drum fills the air. Together, you honor the benevolent Father Sun spirit.

The elders present you with a drink called San Pedro or Huachuma. As you take the first sip, the bitter taste awakens your senses. Unlike Ayahuasca, San Pedro imparts lucidity and focus, grounding you in the present moment while allowing you to perceive both the human world and the divine with remarkable clarity.

A sense of deep peace and unconditional love envelops your being as the three wise elders begin to share their sacred knowledge.

Incas

As the Inca elder begins to weave the tapestry of Inca history, his eyes gleam with a deep, timeless wisdom. He takes you on a journey back through the annals of time, where the Inca civilization reigned in all its splendor.

"In the heart of the Andes," he begins, "our ancestors built a kingdom that stretched from the shimmering Pacific to the boundless Amazon. Our people, the Quechua, revered the land as a living deity, and the mountains were our guardians, bearing secrets that would change the course of history."

With each word, the Inca elder paints a vivid picture of a once-mighty empire, where cities of stone and gold dotted the landscape. He speaks of the breathtaking Machu Picchu, the 'Lost City of the Incas,' perched high in the clouds, a sanctuary of unparalleled beauty and mystery.

"From our ancestors, we inherited a profound understanding of the cosmos and the energies that flow through it," he continues. "We learned to harness the power of the earth, the stars, and the elements. We believed in the great cosmic order, and we understood that our spirits were intricately connected to the universe."

As he delves into the teachings of the Incas, the elder imparts a profound secret—a revelation that transcends time itself. He speaks of the 'Qori Kancha,' the 'Temple of the Sun,' a place where gold and silver were revered not for their material worth, but for their spiritual significance. The Inca Empire was built on the principles of balance and harmony, with the sun as the ultimate symbol of divinity.

"We, the Inca, sought to live in harmony with the earth, the sun, and the moon," he explains. "In our wisdom, we recognized the importance of balance and unity within ourselves and with all of creation."

With a smile, the elder reveals the empowerment—a code passed down through generations, a gift of healing and awakening. This code is a key that unlocks the ancient wisdom of the Inca civilization and the understanding of cosmic energies. As you receive this code, you feel a surge of vitality and a profound connection to the very essence of the universe.

"You, dear one, now carry the healing and awakening of the Incas within you," he says. "This legacy is yours to share with others, to bring balance and harmony to the world. The secrets of our people are not lost to time; they reside within you, ready to be unlocked and bestowed upon those who seek the light of wisdom."

As the Inca elder concludes his tale, you are filled with a sense of auspiciousness and purpose. The wisdom of the Incas is alive within you, a beacon of light that can guide your path and illuminate the journey of those you touch with your newfound knowledge.

Mayas

The Maya elder, draped in vibrant garments that mirror the colors of tropical birds, embarks on a captivating narrative, inviting you to step into the wondrous world of the Maya civilization. With a glint in his eyes, he speaks of a people whose wisdom was as vast as the boundless jungles that cradled their ancient cities.

"In the heart of the Yucatan Peninsula and beyond," he begins, "the Maya built a civilization that thrived for centuries. They were astronomers, architects, and scribes, delving deep into the mysteries of the cosmos."

The elder's storytelling paints a vivid picture of the awe-inspiring city of Tikal, where monumental pyramids pierced the jungle canopy, reaching toward the heavens. He speaks of the enigmatic Chichen Itza, a place where time itself was inscribed in stone.

"Our ancestors," he continues, "possessed a deep understanding of the celestial bodies and their influence on earthly life. They observed the movements of the stars and planets, and from this, they crafted a complex calendar—a key to unlocking the cycles of existence."

As he delves into the teachings of the Maya, the elder imparts a profound secret—a revelation that transcends time. He shares to your soul the concept of the 'Hunab Ku,' the supreme creator and the source of all life. The Mayas understood that every individual was a thread in the cosmic tapestry, connected to the divine through their own unique path.

"The Maya believed that life was a sacred journey," he explains. "They revered the balance between light and dark, day and night. Their wisdom was a testament to the interconnectedness of all living beings."

With a warm smile, the elder reveals the empowerment—a code passed down through the ages, a gift of healing and awakening. This code represents the very essence of the Maya civilization, a bridge to the cosmic energies and the wisdom of the ancients. As you receive this code, you feel a surge of vitality and a profound connection to the vast cosmos.

"You, dear one, now carry the healing and awakening of the Maya within you," he says. "This legacy is yours to share with others, a beacon of light to guide those who seek to navigate the intricacies of existence. The wisdom of the Maya endures in your heart, ready to shine whenever you most need it and to be shared with those who yearn for the knowledge of the ages."

As the Maya elder concludes his tale, you are filled with a sense of profound wisdom and purpose. The heritage of the Maya is alive within you, a testament to the interconnectedness of all life and the sacred journey we all undertake. You carry the keys to this ancient wisdom and the ability to illuminate the path for those you encounter.

Aztecs

The Aztec elder, with regal demeanor and ancient symbols adorning his attire, transports you to the awe-inspiring world of the Aztec civilization. His eyes hold the stories of a people whose history was etched in stone and whose rituals were entwined with the very heartbeat of the earth.

"In the heart of the Valley of Mexico," he begins, "the Aztecs built a civilization that was both powerful and spiritually profound. They believed in the duality of existence, where life and death were inextricably linked, and where their gods were both fierce and nurturing."

The elder's storytelling paints a vivid picture of the magnificent city of Tenochtitlán, set amidst the vast Lake Texcoco. He describes the grandeur of the Templo Mayor, where sacrifices and ceremonies connected the earthly realm to the divine.

"Our ancestors," he continues, "believed in the sacredness of all life. They honored the earth as a giver of sustenance and regarded themselves as stewards of the land. The Aztecs understood that life's greatest gift was to be able to offer oneself in service to the greater whole."

As he delves into the teachings of the Aztecs, the elder imparts a profound secret—a revelation that transcends time itself. He shares the concept of 'Tezcatlipoca,' the deity of fate and the embodiment of change. The Aztecs understood that life was a constant dance of transformation, where death was merely a transition to another state of being.

"The Aztecs believed that the journey of the soul was eternal," he explains. "They revered the balance between life and death, creation and destruction. Their wisdom was a testament to the cyclical nature of existence."

With a compassionate smile, the elder reveals the empowerment—a code passed down through the ages, a gift of healing and awakening. This code represents the very essence of the Aztec civilization, a bridge to the forces of change and the wisdom of the ancients. As you receive this code, you feel a surge of vitality and a profound connection to the eternal cycles of existence.

"You, dear one, now carry the healing and awakening of the Aztecs within you," he says. "This legacy is yours to share with others, a guiding light to those who seek to navigate the ever-changing tides of life. The wisdom of the Aztecs is alive within you, ready to shine whenever needed and to be shared with those who yearn for the knowledge of the eternal dance of creation and destruction."

As the Aztec elder concludes his tale, you are filled with a profound sense of purpose and wisdom. The heritage of the Aztecs resonates within you, a testament to the interconnectedness of all things and the eternal journey of the soul. You carry the keys to this ancient wisdom and the ability to illuminate the path for those you encounter, guiding them through the cycles of creation and transformation.

As the elders conclude their teachings, they share a heartfelt comment with gentle laughter. They reveal that as you dedicate yourself to this path of healing, you may find the path to full awakening. With dedication and commitment, you might even encounter enlightenment in this lifetime, a blessing for yourself and all those you touch with your wisdom.

Surrounded by the sound of the bonfire and the sounds of nature, they point up to the starry sky, and your gaze follows. High above, an eagle and a condor soar gracefully. Their flight is a dance, as if they are the best of friends, united in the boundless sky. As you watch, they transform into pure luminous light, descending to you and entering your heart uniting your heart and mind in perfect balance and union...

A profound sense of love, comfort, and bliss washes over you as you whisper your gratitude for this extraordinary journey. Slowly, you open your eyes and take a deep breath, filled with profound gratitude, celebrating the beauty of this meditation with San Pedro in the sacred mountains of Peru.

- **Shamanic guided meditation with ayahuasca and her Healings: opening the heart, healing emotions, and fixing relationships**

Take a moment to find a quiet and comfortable space where you can fully immerse yourself in this shamanic guided meditation. Sit or lie down, don't need to close your eyes, begin to focus on your breath. Inhale deeply, filling your lungs, and exhale slowly, releasing any tension in your body.

Imagine yourself in the heart of the Amazon rainforest, surrounded by the lush and vibrant colors of the jungle. The air is filled with the sounds of nature—the chirping of birds, the rustling of leaves, and the gentle hum of the river. You are safe and protected in this sacred space.

Now, visualize a circle of shamanic healers and spirit guides forming around you. They are here to support you on your journey with Ayahuasca, the sacred queen of the forest. You can feel their loving and protective energy surrounding you.

As you prepare for this transformative experience, a shaman approaches you with a beautifully adorned cup of Ayahuasca. The cup glistens with the wisdom of the forest, and you accept it with reverence. You can feel the sacred energy of Ayahuasca as you hold the cup in your hands.

Before you take a sip, the shaman invites you to set an intention for your journey. Think about what you wish to heal and transform in your life. It could be about opening your heart, healing your emotions, or mending relationships. Take a moment to clearly state your intention in your mind.

Now, with your intention in your heart, you take a sip of the Ayahuasca. The bitter taste is quickly replaced by a sense of calm and serenity. As the sacred brew begins to work its magic, you can feel a warm, golden light spreading throughout your body.

Ayahuasca takes you on a journey deep within yourself. You may see vivid visions, encounter spirit animals, or experience a profound sense of love and healing. Trust in the process, surrender and let go of any resistance.

Heart opening

With your eyes half open, allow your imagination to transport you to a magical garden within the heart of the Amazon rainforest. This garden is unlike any other, where vibrant and fragrant pink flowers bloom in profusion, their petals glistening like drops of morning dew. These flowers carry the essence of love, and their scent fills the air with an intoxicating sweetness.

As you step into this enchanting oasis, you become aware of the melodious songs of the Amazonian birds, serenading you with harmonious tunes. The energy in this place is palpable, and it surrounds you with a gentle, loving embrace.

This is a sacred space where the wisdom of Ayahuasca and the nurturing presence of the Bobinsana mermaid healers converge. These ethereal beings are guardians of the heart, their energy exuding compassion, kindness, and a deep desire to heal and open the most sacred chamber of your being.

The pink flowers that adorn the garden seem to respond to the call of your presence. Their radiant hues become even more vivid as they sway in the gentle breeze. You approach this symphony of love and are drawn to a particularly resplendent cluster of pink blossoms.

As you reach out to touch them, a rush of warmth and love envelops you, like a cascade of rose petals gently falling around you. You are not alone in this sacred moment. The Bobinsana mermaid healers have arrived, their presence felt as a gentle, aquatic energy that surrounds you, cradling you in their loving embrace.

Their melodious songs intertwine with the wind and bird songs, creating a harmonious chorus of love and healing. It's as if the very air is infused with love and compassion. The heart space within you begins to tingle, and you can feel it gently opening, like a delicate bud unveiling its innermost beauty to the world.

With each breath you take, you draw in the pure, healing energy of the pink flowers and the nurturing essence of the mermaid healers. With each exhale, you release any old wounds, fears, or past hurts that have held your heart captive. It's a moment of profound release and renewal.

The symphony of love in this garden continues to grow. The pink blossoms radiate an ethereal light like a rainbow, and the heartbeat of the Amazon rainforest pulsates through each petal just like the loving purring of a pleased kitty. You sense the pure, boundless love that exists within the heart of the universe itself.

The more you surrender to the love and warmth of this sacred garden, the more your heart blossoms. It's a magnificent transformation, like a rare and exquisite orchid in full bloom. Your heart center opens and expands in bliss, and with each beat, it sends waves of love, compassion, and healing throughout your entire being, as you do so you effortlessly bless all realms of existence.

In the presence of the Bobinsana mermaid healers and the pink flowers, you are free to give and receive love with an open heart. Love is no longer a concept; it's a living force that flows through you, connecting you to all of creation. Your heart is like a radiant sun, and its warmth and light are felt by all who come into your presence.

This sacred journey is a profound gift from Ayahuasca and the Bobinsana mermaid healers. It's a transformation that leaves you deeply loved, your heart fully opened, and your soul singing with joy. Take a few more moments in this garden, basking in the love and warmth that continues to saturate every cell of your being, smell the pink bobinsana flowers and as you do so all of your soul gets purified.

When you are ready, you can begin to return from this heart-centered journey, visualise the sacred garden transforming into pure luminous light and dissolving into your heart. knowing that the love you've experienced will remain with you, guiding your interactions and relationships in a more compassionate and open-hearted way. You are forever connected to the love of the universe and the healing presence of Ayahuasca and the Bobinsana mermaid healers.

Healing Emotions

With your eyes half open, let your spirit journey to a paradise deep within the heart of the Amazon rainforest. Here, nature's enchanting symphony blends seamlessly with the profound wisdom of mother nature and Ayahuasca. You stand at the edge of a serene lagoon, its waters a glistening mirror reflecting the vibrant green canopy of the jungle that surrounds you.

The air is rich with the earthy perfume of the rainforest, and the world seems to breathe with life. A harmonious orchestra of sounds fills the air—the gentle rustle of leaves, the soothing hum of cicadas, and the melodious songs of birds that serenade your soul.

With a graceful step, you wade into the lagoon, the water's tender embrace cooling your skin. A silken mist begins to gather around you, caressing your body with warmth and tenderness. It is the essence of Ayahuasca, a sacred healer, extending an affectionate invitation to become one with its profound magic.

This mist envelops you, like a lover's touch, and as it brushes against your skin, you can feel a profound shift taking place within. It is a healing touch, guiding you on a journey of emotional healing that transcends the ordinary.

You decide to enter this wonderful place, Each step into the lagoon becomes a release, a surrender of all that has burdened your heart. The lagoon embraces you with its tenderness, inviting you to let go of the emotions that have clung to you. It becomes a sanctuary, a cradle of healing, transforming your pain into profound peace and liberation.

The waters hold the wisdom of past, present and future, working in harmony with your being to release emotional traumas and blockages. In this enchanted lagoon, you witness the mirror-like reflection of your emotional healing, a dance of light and shadow unveiling your burdens drifting away.

As you breathe deeply, you feel the emotional release like a gentle rain washing away any sorrow in a form of dark water leaving and being replaced by pure crystalline bright. The jungle around you joins in a soothing serenade, with all the nature spirits of the surroundings, the flower spirits, the trees and the rocks celebrate while holding the space for your healing, and the ripples on the water's surface become a tranquil mirror, reflecting your newfound emotional equilibrium.

In this Edenic haven, you have allowed Ayahuasca and her team to guide you on a journey of emotional healing. Emerging from the water, your heart is lighter and more open, ready to embrace life with renewed emotional strength and resilience.

As you continue your journey, a luminous figure emerges from the lagoon's depths. It is Mother Oshun, the spirit healer of the waters, an embodiment of love and healing. She extends a hand to you, a gesture of profound connection and support and washes your eyes and your heart symbolising purification.

Mother Oshun's loving presence surrounds you as you bask in the soothing waters of the lagoon. Together, you allow the waters to carry away any emotional burdens that no longer serve you. You are free to move forward with a heart that is unburdened and open to the full spectrum of human emotions, like a magnificent songbird that knows no bounds.

Healing Relationships

As you close your eyes, envision yourself in a cosmic realm, far from the confines of Earth, surrounded by celestial beings aglow with radiant blue light. You stand within a magnificent temple of shimmering sapphire and crystal, its ethereal beauty transcending earthly bounds.

The air in this celestial haven is charged with the energy of pure healing and transformation. It fills your being with a sense of serenity and boundless love, connecting you to the very essence of the universe.

In this transcendent space, you are invited to embark on a profound healing journey for your relationships, guided by the wisdom of Ayahuasca. It is a journey of reconciliation and forgiveness, and you hold the ancient healing mantra of Ho'oponopono in your heart—four simple phrases that carry the power of transformation: "I love you, I am sorry, please forgive me, I am grateful."

As you breathe deeply, envision the people in your life who have played a significant role in your journey. They appear one by one, their presence illuminated by the radiant blue beings surrounding you. Feel their presence in your heart and mind.

For each person, repeat the sacred words of Ho'oponopono. "I love you [for the reason....], I am sorry [for the reason....], please forgive me [for this specific words or actions....], I am grateful [for the reason....]." Say these words from the depths of your soul, allowing them to resonate through the vast expanse of this cosmic realm.

As you utter these words, visualize the people you hold in your thoughts responding to your intentions. See their energy softening, their essence filling with understanding, and their hearts opening to receive your healing. Watch as any tension or conflict dissolves, replaced by a sense of reconciliation and love.

As you continue through your list of people, be aware of the emotions that arise within you. The act of repeating these words brings about a profound sense of release and transformation. With each repetition, you are clearing away the barriers that have stood between you and these individuals.

The power of Ho'oponopono, in this celestial realm, is like a gentle cosmic wind, washing away any pain or resentment that has clouded your relationships. It brings clarity, understanding, and a renewed sense of love and gratitude.

As you reach the end of your list, you may find that your heart feels lighter, and a deep sense of peace fills your being. The relationships in your life have been touched by the healing power of forgiveness and love, resonating with the cosmic energies that surround you.

Take a few moments to sit in this space of profound healing and gratitude. Feel the unity and love that now flows between you and those you have healed. You have created a sacred space for reconciliation and harmony in the cosmic realm, and your heart is a vessel of love and understanding.

When you are ready, slowly open your eyes, knowing that you have taken a significant step in healing and nurturing your relationships. The power of Ho'oponopono, guided by the infinite wisdom of your team of spirits, is a profound force for transformation and love in the vast cosmic tapestry of existence.

As your journey continues, the shamanic healers and spirit guides surround you, offering their guidance and support. They are here to assist you in your healing process.

When you are ready, you can begin to return from your journey with Ayahuasca. Take a few deep breaths and feel yourself grounding back into your physical body. Know that the healing you've experienced will continue to work in your life.

Open your eyes, and carry the love, healing, and wisdom of Ayahuasca with you as you move forward in your journey of transformation and growth.

- **A journey together with the Author in one of his favourites Ayahuasca out of body experience**

Once upon a time, in the heart of the Amazon rainforest, the author embarked on a journey that would transcend the boundaries of ordinary reality. It was a night unlike any other, under the canopy of stars and the watchful eyes of the ancient jungle. The Amazon was alive with the songs of unseen creatures, and the air was thick with the wisdom of the rainforest.

As the author partook in an Ayahuasca ceremony, the brew began to work its magic, and the world around him transformed. He found himself on a surreal and enchanting journey that transcended the confines of the physical realm.

The author's consciousness soared into the cosmos, leaving behind the limitations of his earthly vessel. He floated amidst the stars, a celestial being in the tapestry of the universe. The constellations danced in a celestial ballet, and he could feel the harmony of the cosmos coursing through his very essence.

In this astral realm, the author encountered beings of light, radiant and otherworldly. They communicated not through words, but through the language of the heart and soul. It was a conversation beyond the limitations of human speech, an exchange of pure love and wisdom.

These beings guided the author on a journey through the dimensions of existence, revealing the interconnectedness of all life. He witnessed the past, present, and future as threads woven into the cosmic fabric, each action and choice rippling through time and space.

In this surreal odyssey, the author delved into the mysteries of the universe. He learned of the interplay of light and shadow, the dance of creation and destruction. It was a revelation that every experience, no matter how challenging, was a stepping stone on the path of awakening.

As he journeyed deeper into the cosmic tapestry, the author's own consciousness expanded. He realized that he was not separate from the universe but an integral part of it. He felt a profound sense of interconnectedness with all living beings, a tapestry of unity that transcended individuality.

This out-of-body experience was an awakening of the highest order. The author understood that the pursuit of liberation and enlightenment was not a solitary endeavor but a journey of interconnected souls. It was a call to embrace the boundless potential within and to share the light of wisdom and love with others.

In this surreal journey, the author's spirit soared, touching the very essence of existence. He felt a deep sense of purpose and a commitment to the well-being of all beings. It was a journey that left an indelible mark on his soul, a testament to the boundless possibilities of human consciousness.

As the Ayahuasca ceremony drew to a close, the author returned to his earthly vessel, forever changed by the cosmic odyssey. He carried with him the wisdom of the stars, the love of the celestial beings, and a profound understanding of the interconnectedness of all life.

This real-life story serves as a testament to the limitless potential of the human spirit. It inspires us to embark on our own journey of self-discovery and awakening, to pursue the path of liberation and enlightenment not only for our benefit but for the benefit of all living beings. It is a call to transcend the ordinary and embrace the extraordinary, to become a beacon of light and love in a world where kindness and compassion are not luxuries but necessities.

- **Protection and empowerment of the blue macaw, Bobinsana mermaid and the White Eagle in a shamanic transmission that will bless you for a lifetime**

In this sacred shamanic transmission, you find yourself standing on the edge of a serene, shimmering river deep within the heart of the Amazon rainforest. The air is infused with the vibrant energy of the jungle, and the world around you pulsates with life.

Before you, the pristine river stretches into the distance. With a nod, the spirits of the blue macaw, the Bobinsana mermaid, and the White Eagle, your eternal protectors, await you.

As you step into the river's waters, you are instantly transformed into a river-dwelling being, embraced by the spirit of the Bobinsana mermaid. She is a vision of ethereal beauty, with long, flowing hair and a deep connection to the water's wisdom. The Bobinsana mermaid takes your hand and leads you beneath the surface.

Submerged in the river's depths, you encounter a realm of vibrant underwater life. The spirits of the bobinsana transform into the very water that surrounds you and whisper guidance to you as you dive deep within these sacred waters.

You find yourself surrounded by a beautiful cristalyne underwater city. Within a underwater sanctuary, the enlightened spirits of the water converge in a profound shamanic alliance. They channel their energy into your being, fortifying your spirit, and enveloping you in their blessings. The river's waters, now illuminated with their divine light, infuse you with protection and empowerment from the waters giving you the code of water healing and transformations to benefit yourself and others during your healing journey.

As you stand within the grotto, the spirit of the Bobinsana mermaid infuse your being with her sacred energy, blessing you for a lifetime she says those winsdoms will come alive during your ceremonies and on the times of need you will know what to do, just go with the flow and you will be fully guided. Your spirit becomes a radiant beacon of their wisdom, illuminating your path and safeguarding your journey.

As you emerge from the grotto, your spirit glows with the radiant energies of these spirit allies, and the wisdom of the sacred waters infuses your being. Above you, the blue macaw, the Bobinsana mermaid, and the White Eagle joyously welcome you back, celebrating your transformation with jubilant expressions. They perceive the deep purification within your soul, bearing witness to your profound awakening.

In whispered tones, they gently remind you that whenever you partake in Ayahuasca, they will be the first ones to eagerly await your arrival on the other side.

Approaching you is a Shaman, a vessel of boundless wisdom and love. With grace and reverence, he positions his mouth above your head and softly exhales the sacred tobacco smoke, infusing your being with the blessings of the spirits of the blue macaw, the Bobinsana mermaid, and the White Eagle.

Once more, a gentle breath of sacred tobacco smoke ascends above your head as the shaman chants the enchanting words, "Mariri, mariri, mariri, Arcana Grande Espirito." With a tender kiss, he seals this profound connection, his hand resting gently above your head.

From this transformative moment forward, you carry within you the radiant empowerment of the blue macaw, the Bobinsana mermaid, and the White Eagle. Guided by the great spirit himself, your shamanic journey is now brilliantly illuminated with their profound wisdom, unwavering protection, and an endless wellspring of boundless love.

Closing with Gratitude, Trust and Surrender

In closing this transformative journey, let us embrace the profound wisdom that the Amazon, the sacred plants, and the ancestral spirits have shared with us. The healing, the revelations, and the luminous transformations are yours to cherish and carry forward.

With hearts brimming with gratitude, we extend our deepest appreciation to all those who have contributed to this work—both seen and unseen, physical and spiritual. Our reverence extends to the indigenous peoples of the Amazon who have entrusted us with the guardianship of their traditions.

To you, dear reader, who embarked on this odyssey, we offer our profound thanks for your trust and your presence. It is you who breathes life into these words, and it is you who carries the wisdom of these pages into the world.

Ayahuasca teaches us to always remember to trust and surrender as we are always fully guided and deeply loved.

As we part ways, let us remember that the journey is far from over. It is a path that unfolds with each step, inviting us to seek further, to discover more, and to delve deeper into the wellspring of wisdom that flows within us.

The next chapter awaits, dear traveller. And as the final note of this tale, we leave you with the enduring truth that your heart is a vessel of boundless potential, your spirit is a beacon of light, and the universe is conspiring in your favour.

May your journey continue to be one of healing, growth, and profound self-discovery. Until we meet again, under the canopy of stars, in the embrace of nature, or within the sacred chambers of your own heart—farewell, and may your path be eternally illuminated.